Personal Health:

Tired of Tiredness!

How to Overcome Being Tired All the Time and Beat Chronic Fatigue for Life.

(Healthy Living, Healthy Eating & Self Healing)

Sofia Johansson

Disclaimer

This book is intended for informational purposes only. It is not designed to treat, cure, or diagnose any disease, health problem or medical condition, and then it is up to the reader to consult a healthcare professional.

This book is not a substitute for medical advice. The author is not to be held liable for any injury the reader may endures as a result of reading this book.

Sofia Johansson

Table of Contents

Sofia Johansson

Introduction

Thank you and congratulations for downloading the book, "Tired of Tiredness! How to Overcome Being Tired All the Time and Beat Chronic Fatigue for Life."

In this book, you will learn more about tiredness and chronic fatigue. You will become familiar with the signs and symptoms that point to issues of fatigue and the possibilities of where they arise from. You will gain a wider perspective on the habits and lifestyles of both those that contribute to feelings of tiredness as well as those that contribute to a healthier, energetic lifestyle. When you are able to better gauge which activities or non-activities contribute to your fatigue and which ones are energizing, you will be better equipped to make the right decisions every step of the way in living an exhaustion-free life.

Get to learn effective and doctor-recommended techniques to overcome fatigue. Come to know everyday remedies that have stood the test of time over thousands of years that still hold true today. Sometimes all it comes down to is a matter of a few habit changes and developing a healthy mental outlook on life to get you back on the energy boost wagon. In accordance with this kind of mindset, you will also be introduced to different ways of looking at problems, stresses, and ways to cope in life. If you choose to be consistent with them, they will help to strengthen you and cultivate your own power with such endurance that you will wonder why people have not been taught these things from young ages as a part of everyday life and practice.

By the time you are done reading this book, you will have the tools and the knowledge you will need to beat fatigue. Your journey to improving your life begins right after you're done reading, perhaps even as you read this book. It is all a matter of how far you choose to run with it and when you choose to begin.

This is a tortoise versus the hare race, if you should even consider it to be a race, so the most important thing is that you find the pace that is right for you. Too fast and you might become overwhelmed or discouraged. Too slow and you may also become discouraged from the lack of results. At your own pace and with consistency, the small steps add up over time. Soon enough, with patience and practice, the transformation will have occurred within you right under your nose! You will find yourself with more energy and more capable to fill your life with what truly matters to you.

Just remember that this is not a quick fix. That's why so many people are attracted to the "pill" solution for everything, because they want a fix and they want it immediately. The truth is though, it is most often the lifestyle choices that we make that put us in the position we currently find ourselves in. So then, the "quick fix" becomes a temporary solution that we have to keep repeating (and really become dependent upon) so long as our habits and lifestyles remain the same, which is no fix at all. The contents within this book and suggestions for solutions are long term, true fixes. They are not a Band-Aid. They are the potential for an internal cure.

The "long term" means that yes, they take time to fully integrate into your lifestyle, but once they do, they will carry you and continue to give back to you for the rest of your life so long as you maintain them. The "fix" means that you are letting go of habits and choices that work against you and keep holding you back from truly feeling great, while realigning your body and mind to work together as they naturally do, tuning into the generator process that keeps you feeling energized when you need it, and calm but ready at other times.

So if you are prepared, get ready for a transformation within your life. Get ready to begin seeing your life as you truly wish it and allow yourself to remain open to the surprises that life has to offer which are so great you could not have even imagined them for yourself. Wake up to a new beginning with fresh potential in every moment!

Again, congratulations and enjoy!

Chapter 1

Fatigue: The Truth Exposed

A rose by any other name is still a rose. Fatigue, exhaustion, tiredness, listlessness, or lethargy—they all mean one thing; it is a looming lack of energy, whether physical or mental. Over longer periods of time or repetitive short periods of time feeling like this, it can also lead to the loss of motivation and possibly depression; not just in your mind, but in the chemistry of your brain and body too.

Becoming aware of the signs and symptoms, whether they have been ongoing or just beginning, is the first step in relieving yourself from the deluge of tiredness and chronic fatigue. The sooner that you can identify the problem – more specifically, the source of it – the sooner you can remove it from your life entirely. The proposed trouble with diagnosing fatigue symptoms and illnesses is that they can affect people in many different ways, and the seriousness of it can vary greatly. You should note that this book is not intended to diagnose or help you diagnose an illness. If your condition is noticeably affecting your life, you should seek professional help.

By exploring what fatigue is, the many ways it can affect you, possible causes and common, universal solutions to heal, your understanding of this feeling will increase along with your ability to do something about it. This book will see that you are better informed so that you can take more decisive action in your lifestyle. It will help you synchronize the energy levels of your body with your mind. You will learn more about how to distinguish in which way fatigue relates to you, cultivate and sustain heightened levels of energy, and curb that feeling of fatigue to stay right at the edge of your pillow. A lot of times that's exactly where it all starts, even if you think you're getting enough hours and still don't feel rested.

While physical and mental fatigues have different characteristics, they often exist at the same time. Physical fatigue is characterized by the ebbing of the body's normal physical activity levels. On the other hand, mental fatigue gives you a hard time sleeping and you often lose concentration.

It is a Symptom

Please note that fatigue is not a sign, but actually a symptom. How is this so? A symptom is something that you feel, like a headache, while a sign is something that your doctor can see without even asking you about how you feel, like rashes. Fatigue is a non-specific symptom, meaning it is caused by a lot of different things.

Physical Fatigue

Physical fatigue is when your muscles have difficulty doing what they usually do with ease. Have you had trouble going up the stairs lately? How about when carrying something heavy? You are experiencing muscle weakness resulting in minimized strength to perform things that you never had trouble doing before.

Mental Fatigue

Mental fatigue is manifested when you have trouble focusing on something or when you lose your concentration. This may cause disruption of your daily routines. You feel sleepy and weak; you can't even get out of bed. This is can be a debilitating condition that has tragic results, like when you are driving on the freeway and you suddenly lose concentration. You might end up in an accident.

Fatigue Spares No One

Even the strongest can feel fatigue. Experts say about 10% of the global population suffer from fatigue at any given time. In the

United States alone, the National Institute of Health says that one in five people claims to be suffering from fatigue that is severe enough to disrupt their daily activities.

Fatigue and Sleepiness

Fatigue is not the same as sleepiness. Fatigue is a chronic condition and it can be an indication of a medical illness. On the other hand, sleepiness is caused by not having enough sleep and it can be a symptom of a more serious medical condition.

Signs and Symptoms

When you are suffering from fatigue, you feel exhausted after an activity, whether physical or mental. Your feeling of tiredness is not relieved even when you rest or get some sleep. A severe condition may cause a disruption of your normal activities.

A more severe condition is chronic fatigue that is a result of not doing any physical activity but a loss of motivation. Patients diagnosed with clinical depression may complain of chronic fatigue.

The signs and symptoms of fatigue can either be mental, physical, or emotional. If you observe the following signs and symptoms, you might be suffering from fatigue:

Body malaise

Lack of motivation

Dizziness

Headache, especially if in a new pattern

Lack of focus

Hallucinations

Muscle and/or joint pain

Inability to concentrate

Poor short-term memory

Coordination is impaired

Irritability

Impaired judgment

Mood swings

Pain after any activity

Loss of appetite

Sore throat

Enlarged lymph nodes

Drowsiness

Slowed reflexes

Causes

When you take a look at the possible causes of fatigue, the list might go on and on. You can ask medical experts and they will tell you that most illnesses include fatigue or body malaise as a possible symptom. Some of these illnesses to rule out will be provided at the end of this section.

Your lifestyle or your line of work could be the possible cause of your fatigue. Are you a doctor or a nurse? The long hours at work result in irregular sleeping patterns that can make you feel tired all the time. Police officers are also prone to fatigue because their job sometimes entails physical activities, especially those who are assigned to the night shift.

Is there a newborn in the house? This is one cause of a disruption of your sleeping patterns because you often find yourself roused from sleep in the wee hours of the morning.

Do you consume too much coffee during the day? Doing so can lead to sleep problems.

There are drugs and medications like antidepressants and steroids that can cause you to feel tired all the time. Statins can cause extreme tiredness. They are usually prescribed to patients with high levels of cholesterol.

Clinical depression can cause you to feel tired all the time.

Endocrine and metabolic problems like diabetes, hypothyroidism, kidney disease, liver disease and anemia can cause fatigue.

Heart conditions like arrhythmia, congestive heart failure, hypotension and coronary heart disease can cause extreme fatigue that disrupts your daily activities.

Lung problems like pneumonia and asthma are also causative agents of fatigue.

Constant lack or loss of sleep will make your lethargic. Sleep problems like chronic snoring, sleep apnea, and insomnia are causative agents of fatigue that also play into chronic fatigue in some cases.

Infectious diseases (HIV, tuberculosis, and hepatitis) are also leading causes.

Treatments for various medical conditions can cause lethargy and tiredness in patients. Such treatments include chemotherapy and radiation therapy.

Obesity is also considered a cause. Overweight individuals often complain of having difficulty in climbing the stairs and even walking a short distance already renders them out of breath. On the other hand, lack of weight results in impaired muscle strength, causing you to grow tired after doing only light chores.

Sofia Johansson

Chapter 2

Chronic Fatigue Facts

Chronic fatigue syndrome results in persistent exhaustion and tiredness that can affect your daily routines; it is not relieved after sleep. Oftentimes the quality of one's sleep is affected by CFS negatively. It is an ironic case in which a person feels tired constantly, but they cannot get the rest that they so deservingly need. CFS as it is medically known is also referred to as myalgia encephalomyelitis or ME in Europe and Canada, but it actually isn't certain if myalgic encephalomyelitis is the same disease as CFS or not. Myalgia is characterized by muscle pain, while encephalomyitis is the inflammation of your brain and spinal cord.

Medically speaking, doctors and scientists who have studied CFS continue to expand the knowledge about this quiet disease, as it is difficult to trace, affects us in indefinite ways, yet still contends as a large contributor to the problems we face in being able to live a fully functional life. Employers and others do not readily recognize it as a disputable illness that affects our efforts, so that people who must cope with it must press through their obligations and responsibilities without receiving the proper care and attention that they need to reverse the effects.

For this reason, CFS is also called *chronic fatigue immune dysfunction syndrome* or CFIDS so as not to trivialize the illness when its effects can be quite serious and should be considered so. CFS and prolonged fatigue in general deal directly with the immune system, and where one's immune system becomes compromised, more illness is welcomed to set in. This is why it is so important to identify the causes and stamp them out as soon as possible so that your condition does not exacerbate into something even more serious.

CFS is a serious condition and can cause long-term medical disability if it is not taken care of. Anyone, regardless of sex or age, can suffer from CFS, but experts say that is more common among women than in men. This may be a reflection however of simply who reaches out for help more than who is most affected by the disease.

The statistical information is difficult to gather for CFS because it goes underreported, since so many people who have it do not realize it, don't report it to their doctors, or don't see it as a condition and rather have come to accept a meager daily struggle of maintaining energy as regular part of life when it truly isn't. It also doesn't help that we live in a society that demands more of us without making healthier lifestyle choices as readily available as those that deplete us of energy.

Instead, we are conditioned to think that daily fatigue is a regular part of life that everyone must face, so here, let's swill a couple pots of coffee, take a pill or two, and add a small bottle or powdered energy into our drink to keep us going throughout the day. These are all patches – Band-Aids – they are temporary fixes that do not address the problem at its roots, and until that is done, the problem will persist. Then we just become consumers dependent on an insufficient and expensive lifestyle that has been carved out for us, rather than engaging in practices that help us to cultivate our own energy so that we may carve out our own lives as we see fit.

How Life Changes with CFS

Most CFS cases are mild to moderate. However, there are some sufferers who complain of severe symptoms.

o   Mild CFS – You can still take care of yourself but you will need time to rest.

o   Moderate CFS – This is characterized by reduced mobility. You may experience changes in your sleep patterns.

o   Severe CFS – You can do only minimal activities but your mobility is significantly reduced. Concentration is also adversely affected.

The factors can be many and they can also be a combination of things, including but not limited to mentally or emotionally stressful events, endocrine and neurological dysfunction, and others. It has been related to the cause of being infected with the same virus that causes mononucleosis (mono), and this was the leading theory for many years, however after further research it has been shown that not all CFS cases begin with a viral infection. Candida Albicans, an infectious yeast found in the lower intestines that feeds off of sugars and simple carbohydrates in the diet, has been associated with CFS, as well as bacteria-like pathogens, other intestinal viruses and infectious agents.

There have been three central nervous system (brain and the spinal cord) components that appear to be consistent problems for most CFS sufferers:

Hypothalamus-pituitary-adrenal (HPA) axis dysfunction

The hypothalamus is also known as the "master gland" of the body. It controls and regulates the hormone levels in the body that contribute to all of the body's regulated functions; blood-glucose levels, serotonin (happy hormone) levels, cortisol (stress hormone) and derivative levels, sleep patterns, periods of energetic exertion as well as periods of rest and cell regeneration.

The pituitary gland sits just below the hypothalamus in the brain and acts as second in command for hormone production and regulation. Based on information received from various places and organs throughout the body, the hypothalamus secretes primary hormones to keep levels regulated and the pituitary gland sends those hormones along with messages and other secondary hormones to specific places in the body, which need to be regulated.

The adrenal glands sit on top of the kidneys and play a part in affecting our metabolism, but they also directly relate to our stress levels by their secretion of cortisol. These are the glands that have contributed to our "fight or flight" survival response that have kept us alive through evolution. Now that we are living in a stage where this immediate need for survival is no longer pertinent, our brains are left up to dictating the "necessary" amount of adrenal function based on what we perceive as stress and how we react to it. In this day and age, that can relatively be anything under the sun, which actually makes it more dangerous for us because we can be raising our cortisol levels needlessly, keeping our body and mind in a constant state of stress that serves us no purpose and ends up harming us instead. Excess stress and cortisol levels can be seen as a contributing factor to prolonged fatigue to this effect.

HPA axis dysfunction can lead to a sluggish but persistent stress response and eventually to adrenal dysfunction. This dysfunction has also been seen to contribute to depression as well, which again plays into one of the complications of CFS. It all comes down to cortisol secretion. Excessive cortisol secretion, which suppresses serotonin, leads to depression. People with CFS usually have *lower*-than-normal levels of circulating cortisol in the blood.

Neutrally mediated hypotension

What does this mean? Well, *hyper*tension is synonymous with high blood pressure. Blood pressure is a crucial component of your body's health because it is blood that carries all the nutrients from the food you eat and oxygen from the air you breathe into every single cell of your body. Likewise, it is also your blood and circulatory system that carries all of the waste that each cell produces and carbon dioxide back into the kidneys, heart, and lungs so that it can be excreted from the body.

Furthermore, your HPA axis function works directly through the circulatory system because this is how hormones travel throughout the body. Unlike nerve impulses that send messages and monitor body functions instantly, the diffusion of hormones throughout the body via the circulatory system is an ongoing process that takes time to see results. This is why many prescription medications require a few weeks for sustained effects to take place, and why it takes weeks for the rudimentary changes suggested in this book to take effect as well.

Your blood pressure is determined by the strength of your heart muscles, it's regulated rhythm or heartbeat, and the cleanliness of the insides of your blood vessels, whether they are congested or blocked by cholesterol, clots, or other factors. It is also determined by the flexibility of your blood vessels. Certain lifestyle choices such as inadequate daily water intake (consistent, mild dehydration), smoking, and unhealthy eating can all lead to the stiffening of your blood vessels, affecting your overall blood pressure and your overall health. Believe it or not, it is actually better to have high blood pressure rather than low blood pressure. With high blood pressure, strain is placed on the heart and your blood vessels, however with low blood pressure, you actually are not getting enough blood to circulate adequately throughout the body. This can lead to far more serious complications than high blood pressure presents.

Hypotension is synonymous with low blood pressure, and the factor that we're speaking of here in regards to CFS is actually a neurological symptom in which impulses from the brain to the circulatory system do not keep the blood vessels contracted enough to maintain a normal blood pressure. This situation is also connected to an inappropriate response to adrenaline.

Neurotransmitter imbalance

This is one problem of CFS patients that is at the forefront of research on understanding and being able to accurately identify the disease, although it is highly intrusive. Scientists have taken samples of patients' cerebrospinal fluid – that fluid which bathes the brain and brain stem to help keep it cool, maintain its shape, as well as a number of other beneficial factors – and have noticed that people with symptoms of CFS have several proteins in their cerebrospinal fluid that is specific to the disease. It has been noted that this is one of the first consistent biological markers that has been discovered.

What are the Causes of CFS?

Doctors have yet to pinpoint what the exact causes are. As it has been said, it is difficult for doctors to catch and thus far has primarily been diagnosed by ruling out other diseases with a similar profile. It is very important that the appropriate conditions that are present be identified and the ones, which are not present also, since some, may be more serious than CFS. There are some theories that have been formed, other than those mentioned previously, as to the root causes of CFS:

Hormonal imbalance

Infections

Stress

Emotional trauma

Psychological problems

Poor immune system

More studies are needed to determine the exact causes of the condition.

Treatment

There are no specific treatments that target alleviating the symptoms. However, doctors recommend therapy, an exercise program, and medication to address pain and sleeping disorders. Basically any lifestyle choices that can be made to support the body as fully as possible are encouraged by modern physicians to help relieve CFS symptoms.

This means that it will do one well to avoid stress as much as possible – that goes to say any stimulus, emotional or physical, that requires the body to adapt to a strenuous change should be removed from one's life so that they may recuperate properly and effectively. The diet choices one makes are another front from which CFS can be relieved, avoiding stimulants like caffeine, nicotine and sugar as well as depressants like alcohol as much as possible. The exercise one takes up to counter the effects of CFS should be consistent and gentle, within one's tolerance so that problems do not get agitated and become worse.

A crucial part of treatment, as it goes with anything really, is education, since the more that one knows about an issue and problem, the better choices they can make to handle its challenges. So far we have talking about the issues, so let's segue into what those choices look like in a comprehensible lifestyle and how you may feel from doing them too. By observing how others feel from a rudimentary standpoint in feeling a stride throughout the day, fueling themselves in their efforts, you can get an idea of what the better choices are. From there, you will be provided with effective methods to turn to those better choices on a daily basis. Integrate these methods together into your routine on all fronts, in a stepped pace, and the fruits of your efforts will multiply in the wake of your symptoms subsiding. Let's cruise now into how some people seem to have so much energy, regardless of age!

Chapter 3

Why Some People Have More Energy than Others

There are people who get what they want and there are those who don't. The latter have this very glaring difference: energy! Yes, you read it right. It's neither your ability nor your intelligence that propels you to succeed, but how much energy you have!

Here's why: you may be intelligent but without the energy to act, then your intelligence is useless. When you have the best abilities but you don't have energy, your abilities don't mean anything.

Did you know that there is an energy crisis all over the world? Millions of people around the globe have "fossil fuels." People these days get up in the morning thinking about the enormous tasks that need to be done for the day and they feel exhausted already. Still, some consider these tasks as challenges.

Emotional Energy

So why do some people have more energy than others? Experts say that most people lack emotional energy rather than physical energy. Emotional energy is the aliveness of the mind and the spirit that keeps you connected to the vitality of life. It is having that sense of being happy, resilient, and being open to whatever challenges life gives you. People who have high emotional energy are more loving. They easily rise above difficult situations. They do not have a problem in making decisions that are potentially life-changing.

Emotional Fatigue

People work too hard to make a living. There are family obligations to fulfill. There are emergencies and problems that can render most people powerless and hopeless. It therefore doesn't really come as a surprise that most people feel tired, but most of the time, this extreme exhaustion can be classified as emotional fatigue.

You have learned about physical and mental fatigue, but what is emotional fatigue? It is another form of fatigue, but this time, utter exhaustion is brought about by tiredness of the spirit. Physical energy is dependent on your age, mental fatigue starts with the mind, whereas emotional energy has little to do with your upbringing.

You may be physically and mentally tired, but emotional energy can change everything.

Physical and Emotional Energy

Physical energy is limited while emotional energy is not. As your body ages, your physical strength and energy diminish, but you can make emotional energy work for you. Once you enhance your emotional energy, your hopes and dreams will just be within your reach.

It is one thing to just get through the day and it is another to feel fulfilled for what you were able to accomplish. The difference between them is emotional energy. It is actually hard to tell whether what you are feeling is emotional or physical fatigue, but just the same, you still have to drag yourself in order to do what is expected of you (though it may feel like a burden on your part).

Emotional fatigue can be likened to mental fatigue because you feel exhaustion from the inside. No matter how much you sleep or change your eating habits, you are still extremely exhausted.

Why Do You Need to Boost Your Emotional Energy?

Emotional energy gives you what you need to make an effort to do something. Picture this: you wake up in the morning and you still feel dead tired despite getting a decent sleep, but you still find it in you to drag yourself out of bed because you have a lot of things to do. This is exactly what emotional energy is all about.

The answer to the question why some people have more energy and others do not is found in the successive paragraphs:

ü   People with high energy make it a point to do something new every so often. When your body gets used to the routines, your "fire" to live is slowly extinguished. It's like having a small hole in a water tank that slowly spills water out until you have no more. Excite yourself sometimes. Do or try something new. Even a change in the route you usually travel to and from work is a welcome change. This is just one of the things that energetic people practice.

ü   Those who are bursting with energy are still in touch with their reason for living. They haven't lost their enthusiasm to do what they love the most. Their life's meaning is their very reason for living. This is what keeps them going despite the challenges.

ü   They do not dwell on their past regrets and make it an effort not to live in the past. The feelings of resentment, guilt, and regret over past mistakes, missed opportunities, and heartbreaks rob you of the opportunity to enjoy the present. Energetic people believe that they don't own all the problems and the disappointments in the world so they stop feeling sorry for themselves. They left the past where it belongs and they are living the moment. Dwelling on the past robs you of the needed energy you need to seize the day—the *present* day.

ü   Energetic people keep their "flywheel" spinning. A flywheel is a mechanical device that stores energy which gives you fuel when you need it. For people, it is a passion for something. People bursting with energy keep their flywheels burning and spinning. Find your passion and find something that you are most interested in and pursue it. A hobby ensures that you do not get lost in the monotony of your daily routines.

ü   It can be as simple as jogging around the neighborhood or riding a bicycle. Maybe there is something that you want to collect. Why not start collecting something that you are most interested in like mugs or angel figurines? The idea is to have something that diverts your energy to avoid exhaustion.

ü   Energetic people do not find it difficult to make decisions about anything. When you are trying to decide on something, do not dwell too much on your options. Simply think about the options and decide. The more you dwell on them, the more difficult it will be for you to decide. The agony of finding answers robs you of precious energy. Instead of analyzing, make a good decision. Work on it. You will not know how good or bad a decision will be unless you have decided and acted on it.

ü   Energetic people have the habit of sharing what they have. You hear time and again that the more you give, the more you are given in return. This is what energetic people believe in.

Sofia Johansson

Chapter 4

Beat Tiredness Once and For All

There is no quick fix in beating any form of fatigue. It is a long process but it is doable. It will require a lot of commitment on your part to restore your vitality, but you need not worry because there are a lot of effective ways to beat tiredness.

You have learned how fatigue develops and its different forms. Here are some tried and tested approaches to overcoming fatigue.

Start Consulting Your Doctor

Fatigue can be a sign of a more serious condition. Hence, when you begin to feel extreme exhaustion, you need to visit your doctor regularly. It can be an indication of something serious or it may simply be a case of being burned out, but you do not know that for sure (at least not yet). A visit to the doctor ensures that you are given a proper diagnosis and treatment.

Take Care of Your Body to Beat Tiredness

Watch what you eat

It is important that you make it a habit to eat healthy. If you are tired all the time, change your eating habits and drink at least 10 glasses of water a day. Experts say that even if you eat a well-balanced diet and get enough sleep, you'd still end up tired at the end of each day, hence the recommendation to drink more water. There is research that says when you are tired chronically, you are dehydrated and dehydration is a great energy "zapper."

Taking care of your body also involves performing exercise routines. You need to be active because inactivity contributes to fatigue. Why is this so? You don't use your body much so you don't burn calories that are converted into fuel, so make sure you exercise. You don't need to go to the gym regularly. If you are busy with work and you cannot afford a gym membership, you can try simple activities like brisk walking and jogging. Expose yourself to some early morning sunshine for a full-blown dose of energy and Vitamin D.

Free your mind from internal habits that are sucking the energy out of you.

There is a teaching in Buddhism about mindfulness. It is the practice of appreciating and focusing only on the present moment. It teaches that you shouldn't think about past mistakes because they have long been gone. The only thing that's keeping them alive is your belief in them. If others are hanging onto the past with regard to you, that is their own concern that may be holding them back, but it does not have to be yours. There is something to be said about carrying your own torch and being consistent in your words and actions.

If you have made significant changes for yourself or something from the past simply no longer applies to you, focus only on the consistency and drive of your new endeavors. Old stories and instances that others hold onto about you will fall away like shedding skin because you have become the example of something else now; you are the example of being true to yourself by investing in yourself. Your dedication to feeling energized and cultivating sustained levels of buoyant energy will speak louder than words or any past moment and will define your reality henceforth. All you have to do is keep up with it at your own pace.

On the other hand, the future is about to happen so why do you have to worry about it at the moment? The key to the success of mindfulness is to focus on the "now." Even during the simplest of routines, you can condition your mind. For example, you are walking along a familiar path going to the office. You can start appreciating the sunshine and feel it as it touches your skin. Notice a tree or building that you hadn't recognized before. Take in the colors, textures and smells. Say "hi" to the people who are walking along with you. Chances are they are the very same people that walk with you for the longest time but you just failed to take notice of them. Feel every step as your feet walk on the ground. Appreciate everything!

Watch your life change as you practice this. Your workload won't go away when you keep thinking about it while you're on your way to the office, right? Nor does a utility bill pay itself if you worry about how you will pay for it.

Make that mindset shift fast and you'll feel refreshed even during the most trying times.

Do not dwell on your emotions, especially the negatives

Emotions are very contagious. Have you ever encountered a person who rants about how miserable his or her life is and then you suddenly imbibe the emotions? You then start feeling negative towards everything as well. How about when a friend just cannot stop talking about a blessing or something that made him or her happy? How would you feel? Won't you share their happiness and feel happy, too? That's how contagious emotions can be. So, what do you do? Make evaluations as well as an inventory of the people in your life.

As much as possible, keep away from miserable people because they will just drain you and you end up exhausted. Would you like to know why the vampire craze in media has taken on such popularity? These creatures aren't as fantastical or mythical as they may seem. They are real people who are energy vampires out there and even may have the best of intentions, but because of their corrosive attitudes or lack of effort to take responsibility for their actions, they end up draining the people around them of energy.

These people need to be around the liveliness and energy of others in order for themselves to feel energized, yet they do not generate any from themselves, so they then become a siphon upon the vitality of others and it becomes exhausting. Take the initiative to spend more time with friends who are frequently seeing the positive side of things. Soon enough, you feel as happy as they are, you become motivated, and you get out of that chronic fatigue problem.

Are you a working mom? Chances are you are feeling tired all the time because of the household chores you need to do aside from your responsibilities at work. Please take note, though, that there are working moms out there who can perform their home and office duties without feeling exhausted. It all boils down to how you deal with pressure and stress. Again, negativity sucks the energy out of you so you better practice some mind cleansing and refocusing activities to keep you in the proper perspective. This is where practicing grounding methods to keep yourself balanced really becomes effective and helpful.

A spiritual renewal can benefit you

Once you've decided that you are going to make changes, you have to ensure that you do not lose your focus. Making changes does not necessarily mean that you won't be encountering challenges. You will still encounter them, but this time you'll be more emotionally, physically, and mentally equipped. A spiritual renewal will help keep your mind focused and calm.

A spiritual renewal helps you fight stress, or rather let go of it and anything that may contribute to it, because fighting only creates more struggle and therefore more exhaustion. Meditation is also a good technique to fight the stress that's causing your feeling of exhaustion. When you are able to let go of stress, you don't feel pressured in the things you do, so you are more relaxed.

Yoga is also a good option and it helps you lose weight.

Get enough sleep

Sleep deprivation contributes to fatigue. Sleep restores your strength as it allows your body to relax and heal itself from a day of hard work. It rejuvenates you. However, there are a few things to consider so you can get a more restful sleep. If you want to get the best out of a restful sleep, it is important that you do not eat big meals at dinner time. Take light meals instead; these will be easily digested so you don't have to sleep feeling full. Also, make sure that you eat your meal at least two hours before going to bed, that way you give your digestive system enough time to do its job properly. Avoid drinking caffeinated drinks towards bedtime; you can just drink hot milk as it helps calm you so you sleep better.

Do not turn on the TV right before bedtime. It would be best if you do not place a television set in your bedroom so you can utilize the area just for sleeping and resting. Try reading a book instead.

If you can, consider going to bed earlier so you can also wake up earlier. It also helps to sleep at the same time every night and wake up at the same time, as well. This builds a pattern that your body clock can adapt to.

Exercise regularly

There are a lot of benefits to exercising regularly. It boosts your energy, it helps you get a restful sleep, and it helps you maintain your ideal weight. It also helps you with your balance and flexibility. Make it a habit to jog or brisk walk every morning and do a little stretching. Do not exercise in the evening; you won't be able to sleep easily because of the energy rush.

Step out into the sun

Doctors say that sunlight is still the best stress-buster. You are feeling tired because you are stressed out with so many duties and responsibilities you face on a daily basis. Sunlight is an excellent source of Vitamin D. You don't need to stay too long in the sun, though, especially with the threat of sunspots. A 30-minute walk every morning, preferably before 10 AM, would suffice.

Maintain your ideal weight

Obesity plays a huge role in being lethargic all the time. When you are overweight, it is hard for you to move around so you get less exercise. It also gets in the way of your sleeping patterns. You have low energy so you cannot fight fatigue too well. When you have low energy, you are more inclined to just sit around so you gain more weight, making things worse.

Lose those excess pounds and turn those calories into energy. Cut down on the sweets. Get more exercise.

Get regular massages

Your body needs detoxifying. When you are physically tired, your muscles and joints feel sore. Stress often manifests as body aches and lethargy. Relax and rejuvenate regularly. You can get a massage at least twice a month. Body massages and aromatherapy offered by salons and spas will benefit you tremendously.

The essential oils used during massages send chemical messages to your brain that helps calm you so you become more relaxed.

Go easy on yourself

Sure, you have a lot of duties and responsibilities, but you also have to make sure that you take some rest. You don't have to do it all at once. Prioritize the things that need to be done so it won't be too hard for you. It is more difficult if you put a lot of things on your plate. There's nothing wrong with having to work hard for the family but preserving your health is just as important.

Sofia Johansson

Chapter 5

Putting Energizing Methods to Practice

Now that you have an auspicious direction to lean toward when you are having a moment of doubt or insecurity for what action you should take next, the following methods and exercises are going to provide your filler time with specific steps to take that will help to energize you, encourage a clear mind, and give your confidence a substantial boost among many other benefits.

These exercises may even seem trivial because of how basic they are. It all goes back to some of the very first things we learned when entering into this world: breathing, posture, body mechanics, plus a fresh perspective and approach on just what makes us up and how we can use that knowledge to gain a better control of ourselves. When we can control our actions through treating our body well and making the decisions that will do us the most good, we feel more secure within ourselves. Our judgment becomes better. Our moods stabilize and float on self-satisfaction and contentment. Our capabilities to think clearly and do more increase and we feel more at ease.

We are no longer dis-eased, or taken out of a state of ease, when we make the right decisions to treat our bodies well. We must realize that for as much toxicity in the air, in our food, and in the areas of our life characterized by stagnancy and clutter or overworking, we allow ourselves to tolerate so much while we are still sensitive beings. We have just numbed ourselves to the pain. When we do that we feel less so that we can try to do more, but it's not conducive to our nature. We start to suffer in other ways from mental and emotional exhaustion to spiritual and emotional repression, and/or the eventual onset of physical ailments. Fatigue is therefore a great factor of such lifestyles.

So then, by revisiting the basics and relearning how to form a standard routine of living, we recreate a new standard of living for ourselves that is able to meet and propel our aspirations for what we want out of life. At the very least, it provides us with ample energy to enjoy and appreciate everything that we have going for our lives at this moment.

Breathing Exercises

In the next chapter on eating your way to a healthy body, you will learn about the body's pH levels and how an acidic environment in the body based on what we eat and drink makes fertile ground for bacteria, pathogens and other illness-causing circumstances to thrive. On the other hand, an alkaline environment in the body does not allow for such disease-causing agents to survive.

Did you know though that excessive carbon dioxide and low levels of oxygen in the body also contribute to an acidic environment? On a more basic understanding of oxygen and blood in the body than that, our bodies' cells cannot live without oxygen. We cannot function properly without it. So if we aren't getting enough oxygen into the body by breathing properly and fully, chances are we are going to feel depleted of energy quite often. It has also been noted that people who are overweight, despite their efforts to eat healthy and commit to some form of exercise, still have trouble losing weight and the reason they retain it is because of their poor breathing habits. Shallow breathing is a common factor that does not get enough oxygen into the body. When your cells don't get enough oxygen, they become lethargic. Your metabolism slows down, and therefore you tend to hold onto weight more.

By improving your breathing habits, not only will you be encouraging your cells to work more harmoniously, you will be getting more oxygen to the brain, which will help to clear any mental cloudiness or confusion. You will also feel calmer in state of mind and state of being. Feelings of nervousness, anxiety, and depression will wane over time. You will also be able to get a better rest at night.

It all begins with breathing from the diaphragm. This is the horizontal, circular muscle that sits just beneath the lungs at the bottom of your ribcage. It is located between the rib cage and your upper abdomen, so when you breathe in through the diaphragm, your upper belly should raise. When you exhale, you are simply letting go of the air that has filled your lungs, the diaphragm relaxes, and your upper belly goes back down. This is how you know that you are breathing correctly.

The standard method of breathing that is recommended is by inhaling through the nose and exhaling through the mouth. Some of these exercises will ask you to try different breathing methods. It is good to get a wide-range of experience in because each method serves a certain purpose, bringing attention to different parts of your airways, and when you become more sensitive to the subtleties of them you will feel those effects.

Now then, listed below are some very effective breathing exercises for you to practice. They do not typically take a long time to get the benefits from them so that you can do them in short stints if need be. You can also always extend the period of time that you take to practice them if you so wish. The more you do it, the better.

Breathing Exercise #1:

Find a place where you can sit comfortably with little to no distractions.

Start breathing in through your nose and exhaling through your mouth at the regular pace that you normally breathe.

Focus on your solar plexus (upper belly) expanding with every inhale and deflating with every exhale.

Start focusing on deepening your breaths and developing a rhythmic pace so that the length of your inhales and exhales are equal.

After doing that for a couple of minutes, you will start to notice what areas of your body are holding tension because they will feel tight. Oftentimes these areas are found at the forehead, the number one area for where stress accumulates, which sits right in front of the mind.

If you're having trouble thinking of exactly what you want to say or solving problems most of the time, chances are your thought process could be held uptight, reflected by the tension in your forehead.

Other places where stress and tension commonly accumulate are around the nose, which would reduce the quality of your breathing, as well as the back of the neck, the throat and jaw. The chest and back are other areas where stress accumulates and hinders your capacity to breathe deeply and fully.

When you are breathing during this exercise and begin to notice the areas in your body that are holding tension, place your focus on these areas, one at a time, and "breathe into them".

That is, hold your focus on a particular area in your body, and during your inhalations, imagine that the fresh air is going directly into this place to fill it with healthy oxygen and blood. Essentially that is what the body will do.

The body listens to what the mind tells it on subconscious levels. That's how we accumulate stress from the mental to the physical, and *in reverse*, that's how we can use these exercises to get rid of it. The mind is that powerful. And once you learn how to operate on these subtler levels, you can use your mind to do amazing things – with your body and otherwise.

Continue to breathe deeply in a steady pace, breathing from the diaphragm, expanding and deflating your belly, and "breathing into" the various places of tension in your body, one at a time.

You can do this exercise for 15 to 20 minutes, but at least for 5 to 10 minutes in your day, whenever you have a short break. The more, the better. Focus only on your breath and the areas of tension in the body during this time.

You can always go back to the thoughts of what else is important in your day after you're finished; they'll still be there. Dedicate yourself fully to the moment when you're practicing so that you get all it has to offer. The more you practice, the easier it will be come.

Breathing Exercise #2

This exercise will train you to hold air in from your diaphragm and release it fluidly. Many people when holding their breath tend to hold it in their chest or throat, tightening those muscles and cutting off their natural flow. By holding air in from your diaphragm, the rest of your muscles will be relaxed.

This exercise sees a lot of variants among people who teach it. The method is the same but the increments of time differ. I'll provide you with two common variations here. It will take a little getting used to. From that point if you still haven't found a pace that suits you, you can go online to search for other variations of different time increments or experiment with them yourself.

The first pattern is: 4-2-6-2

This means that you will inhale for 4 seconds from your diaphragm, hold your breath from your diaphragm for 2 seconds, exhale steadily for 6 seconds by relaxing your diaphragm then hold your diaphragm here at the bottom of your exhale for 2 seconds.

Repeat this pattern for a minimum of 5 minutes, going as long as you'd like. Your focus should be on your diaphragm, counting the seconds, and smooth transitions from the holds to the breaths.

If you're holding your breath anywhere but your diaphragm, your exhale will sound like bursts of air releasing from a valve under high pressure. What you should be looking for is a steady flow like the movement of hanging scales going back and forth. In other words, just smooth movements from one direction to another.

You will start to feel it in your abdomen after some time, and perhaps at first 5 minutes of this patterned breathing is all you can do. That's fine. Take breaks to do other things then come back to it. Stick with it, you'll notice results in no time and progress quickly.

Another pattern is all 3's:

Inhale for 3 seconds, hold for 3 seconds at the top of the inhale, exhale for 3 seconds, hold for 3 seconds at the bottom of the exhale. Repeat.

While the first pattern caters a bit more to the way we normally breathe, this pattern of 3's will bring your focus and attention much closer into the breathing and working your diaphragm. Because the increments are shorter, there is a lot more movement going on. It's like the jogging version of breathing exercises.

Because these increments are so short, it does not necessarily mean that you will be taking in full, complete breaths every time. They do not need to be power breaths. Inhale at your regular pace at first rather than trying to inhale to full lungs within 3 seconds every time.

Breathing Exercise #3:

This exercise is designed to really open up the airways in your nasal passages and head. You'll be relaxing the muscles behind your sinuses. When people have colds or sound nasally and stuffed up it's because their sinuses are filled with fluid and/or the muscles surrounding them are tightened or swollen.

This method is very simple.

Start by finding a comfortable place to sit with little to no distractions.

Using the pad of your thumb, cover your right nostril.

Inhale deeply through your left nostril, then use your diaphragm to hold your breath for a moment.

Cover your thumb over your left nostril now and exhale through the right nostril.

Repeat this process for as long as you can, up to 5 minutes.

You may find that this exercise is difficult to sustain at first, especially if you are already experiencing some facial congestion. In fact, it's not recommended that you try this if you do have congestion.

Otherwise, it's a simple starting point that your nasal and facial airways leading down into your throat need to take time getting used to. It could be that they are constricted, especially if you are used to breathing through your mouth. That's perfectly normal, just give it time.

By practicing this method consistently, even if for just short periods at a time, you will be encouraging your body's entire airway system to clear and expand.

Grounding Exercises

In order to get around in this world, everything must start from the ground up. It is where we come from and it is where we go back to, so it might as well be where we build ourselves from in order to reach a healthily energized and sustained state of living. After finding a stable place to build our own world from, we must lay the foundation with encouraging elements and practices that will always nourish us when we come back to them. It is starting from this vantage point how we come to stay fueled and get so much done, feeling so good throughout the day.

When it comes to the body, part of that foundation involves good posture. Poor posture can lead to strained muscles, poor circulation in certain areas, tense joints, and poor breathing habits. It is also a transparent reflection of low self-esteem. Good posture poses to practice can be borrowed from some yoga poses, although these are common to some of our body's natural positions: mountain pose, lotus or cross-legged sitting position, and the Vajra pose, which entails kneeling down and sitting back on your heels while the tops of your feet lay flat on the ground.

Exercise 1:

Relaxing your body and standing straight can also help. Here is a simple exercise you can do anytime, anywhere to open up your hips, build strength in your base, and adequately open up the root chakra, which epitomizes a state of being grounded and will be discussed further next: keep your feet wider than shoulder-length apart and bend your knees a little bit, thrusting your lower body forward gently and tilting the bottom of the pelvis forward. You can hold your hands out in front of you to maintain balance if you need to. Hold this position for a few minutes and then come out of it.

Exercise 2:

This is known as the "Wu Wei" stance from Tai Chi, which is another highly beneficial practice for nourishing healthy movement in the body, promoting relaxed muscles, improved circulation, ease on the joints, and more. This is a stance to remind yourself to get into whenever you are standing on your feet – whether you are waiting in line some place, going out for a walk and resting, or just being social around a circle of friends.

The Tai Chi practice is rooted in Taoism, whose foundational belief is that everything should be done according to how it was naturally designed to do, then learning how to work with our natural design to improve our state of being. So the Wu Wei stance will look completely normal as a regular person standing up. The difference is that you will feel so much better in the bottoms of your feet, your knees, legs, and lower back, and you will be grounded, feeling secure in your stance.

Start by standing with your feet pointing forward, standing directly under your hips. Your knees should be over the tops of your feet and your hips should be facing squarely forward. Get a little bend in your knees and now tilt the bottom of your pelvis forward so that your lower back lengthens out a bit. You should feel the weight of your body in your thighs. Staying in this position, try to lean forward just a bit. Then try leaning back just a bit. You will notice that if you lean forward too much you will start to feel tension in your calves, and if you lean backward too much, you will feel the tension in your shins. The idea is to bring all of that tension snugly into the flexion of your thighs by way of the bend in your knees and the tilt in your pelvis. This will help you to find your correct posture to straighten out the spine. Keep your head up and straight forward. Drop your shoulders and keep your hands and your sides. Breathe from the diaphragm. Stay here for a few minutes and feel the connection of your feet with the ground.

Understanding the Body as an Energetic System

We are marvelous living beings when it comes right down to it, because there is so much that goes into us and flows through us. Everyone is familiar with themselves as a body and the organs, blood, brain and such that make it up. It is not even going out on a limb too much to consider that we are also an intangible thing we call a mind that is capable of extraordinary feats when we put it toward a focused intention. Even though emotions are something that many people either perhaps feel too much or others would rather not even acknowledge, they are a part of our makeup as well. And then there is the notion of spirit, which is difficult for many to define accurately, and varies in opinion from one to the next. Some people have no opinion of such notions.

One certain aspect of us that often gets overlooked in this milieu of our composite is the energetic aspect, even though we're used to talking about having or not having energy all the time! There is an actual functioning, sophisticated energetic system within each and every one of us that has been studied and researched for thousands of years. The western scientific community is beginning to acknowledge its presence, but even so, it exists with or without their acknowledgement. The Ayurveda holistic system of India and the holistic system of Traditional Chinese Medicine are two, several-thousand-year-old systems that give great insight into this intrinsic energetic system of ours, even if they come from differing yet complimentary perspectives.

We will explore the chakra system originating out of India here and see how each chakra associates with particular aspects of our being, what they look like out of balance and one method of how we may work with them to improve the condition of these associations made with them. Chakras are simply energy centers in the body. They relate to the different energies produced by specific organs in the body, energies that relate to emotions, as well as those that relate to aspects of our personalities. By knowing what each chakra relates to, we can determine where we should place our attention in comparison with recognizing how we are feeling and what areas of our lives may need that attention.

At the bottom of each chakra description, you will find vocal exercises that you can practice to help activate and energize these chakras, amplifying their qualities. These exercises involve the same setup as the breathing exercises; finding a nice, quiet place to sit and so on. They also provide pronunciation techniques, as these are important. The wider and more open you can be from your diaphragm up through your chest, neck and mouth, the better. Upon the "m" part, the sound should come out more like the "ng" in "king", creating a vibration in your body that starts from the mouth and reverberates through your cells and bones, eventually working to feel it throughout your body. This has very cleansing effects for the body, stimulating and relaxing effects for the nervous system, and energizing effects for your body as a whole. You will feel lighter afterwards.

Just like we can say that the brain is a muscle that needs to be exercised so that it can function well for you, the same can be said about the chakras. The only difference is how you notice the results. Since the energetic system is one that essentially permeates every aspect of our lives, the results begin very subtly and build upon each other in that way over long amounts of time.

A typical reaction for someone who has been working with their chakra for a month would be the same as a person who just starts jogging for 30 minutes every day without thinking about the results. At the end of that month, you will just take a look at yourself, make a note of how you have been feeling overall, and how much more capable you feel, and you will surprise yourself! Wow! Keep this process in mind when working with this subtle energy system, and trust the process. You will be grateful that you did.

The Root Chakra

Location in the body: At the base of the spine in the tailbone region, between the anus and the external genitalia. This area is also known as the perineum.

Color: Red.

Physical associations in the body: feet, legs, large intestine, bones, spinal column and teeth.

Personality aspects: practicality, courageousness, innocence.

Emotional associations: fear and anxiety, predominantly felt when this chakra is out of balance. Feelings of stability and security when open and healthy. Involves feelings of being grounded with a sense of orientation in the direction of your life, your goals and ambitions.

Mental associations: materialism and attachment to physical things, objects, and money. Also deals with being organized and structured to sort through multiple tasks and to-do lists, being able to prioritize effectively and manage your time well.

An overactive root chakra cause one to become overly materialistic. One can also feel afraid or overly promiscuous. One can also feel excessively insecure and afraid for one's life. Keep this chakra healthy and balanced by going out for a walk every morning and strengthen your body with some regular exercise.

Even a simple jog would do. All of the yoga asanas provided in this book will help you to balance out this chakra most effectively as well, especially the hip opener exercises.

To chant with the root chakra, sit on the ground with legs crossed and hands extended, turned up and resting them on your respective knees. You can keep your palms open or you can touch the tip of the thumb with the index finger, both ways work. It is just about getting focused and calm. Imagine your root chakra at the base of your spine and concentrate on it. As you do this, you will start to feel relaxed. If you want, you can also envision a flower at the chakra that represents the energy blossoming from it. Take deep breaths and do this for a while. You will feel energized and refreshed.

The chant for the root chakra is Lam, pronounced, "Lah-mmm". You can say it with the full extent of each exhale, keeping your throat, neck and chest as relaxed as possible.

The Sacral Chakra

Location in the body: a few inches below the naval in the sacrum area, between the (tops of the) hips.

Color: orange.

Physical associations in the body: pelvic area, lower back, sex organs, sexual energy, kidneys, bladder and fluid functions of the body.

Personality aspects: creativity, awareness, attentiveness, ability to be in the moment.

Emotional associations: sexuality, sensuality, inspiration.

Mental associations: pure knowledge, releases stress, generation of creativity in projects, work, problem solving, and relationships.

This chakra is really important for your creativity and emotions. Problems with the sacral chakra can cause you to be really introverted or really emotional and sensitive. You might start doubting yourself at every step and lose confidence. Feeling intimidated by others and doubting your self-worth is also common. It can also cause confusion with your sexuality and other problems, causing relationship problems in turn.

To open the sacral chakra, you have to sit on your knees in a relaxed position. In yoga, you will know that this position is also known as the Vajra asana. It is really good for your digestive system and your lower body. When you are in this position, extend your hands and fingers open with your palms facing upward. Keep them at your lower midsection, hanging comfortably from your arms, just below the naval where your sacral chakra is. Place your left hand underneath your right hand so that the left can support and the right can direct your energy upward. Try and envision the sacral chakra in your body. If you can imagine a glowing ball of energy, orange in color, that is even better. Breathe out through your nostrils only. You will start to feel relaxed soon.

The chant for the sacral chakra is Vam, pronounced open and deeply as "Vow-mmm".

The Naval Chakra

Location in the body: a few inches above the naval and just below the diaphragm under the rib cage.

Color: yellow.

Physical associations in the body: liver, pancreas, stomach, gall bladder, spleen, digestive system, muscles, lower back and the autonomic nervous system.

Personality aspects: confidence, self-esteem, assertiveness, adaptability and transformation

Emotional associations: source of confidence, assertiveness, playfulness, good sense of humor and emotional transformer that helps you balance the emotions you feel and exert yourself consciously in accordance with them without being carried away.

Mental associations: responsibility for your actions and words, being reliable and stable for yourself and others, ability to meet and take on challenges, being in control of yourself and your life.

Naval chakra imbalances cause you to doubt yourself and give in to others' manipulations easily. Low self-worth and low self-esteem are also common, and introversion is also an effect. Greed, dishonesty, depression, aggression, unnecessary ego, overconfidence, and escapism can also be seen in some people as a result of naval chakra imbalances.

To heal this chakra, you have to sit with your back straight and your knees folded in the Vajra asana position, just like in the sacral chakra section. Bend your elbows and keep your hands in front of your abdomen, above the naval and just below your diaphragm. Rest the heels of your palms on your stomach at the wrist and extend your fingers so that the tips are touching and pointing straight out in front of you. Cross your thumbs, right over left. Close your eyes. You will start to feel calm and composed soon. Do this for a few minutes every day.

The chant for the solar plexus chakra is Ram, pronounced deeply and openly as, "Raw-mm".

The Heart Chakra

Location in the body: middle of the chest, behind the breastbone.

Color: green.

Physical associations in the body: heart, lower lungs, blood and circulatory system, breasts, upper back and thymus.

Personality aspects: houses a person's spirit or true self when there are no mental or emotional burdens weighing on them. Provides the ability to be open and establish well-founded relationships of all kinds, from acquaintances to best friends and loved ones, ability to love and be loved, outgoing, warm, and interactive with others.

Emotional associations: Deals with love, affections, compassion, sense of worthiness, honor, and respect to yourself and others. Also involves feelings of joy, heartache and misunderstanding. As the heart chakra opens, these negative feelings dissolve and you start establishing a relationship with your true self, able to hear it within yourself more often and thereby act on it when thinking and making choices.

Mental associations: deep sense of wellness, self-control and balance. Gives a devotion to think, act and speak without bias towards anyone. Governs and eliminates self-criticism and criticism of others when open.

We have always heard that the heart deals with the matters of love and compassion. Well, that is true. The heart chakra is close to the heart and it is responsible for our emotions of love and affection. It is also responsible for our feelings of fear, heartbreak, and kindness. Many of us are confused as to what true love is or misinterpret it, and there is good reason, because many of the songs and stories that we hear or see about love are actually depicting infatuation or desperation in love, even if they seem sweet. True love has no attachment or need – it generates from within. It gives without expecting a return. It accepts and receives with appreciation and gratitude. It is unconditional. If your heart chakra is blocked you will not be able to express your feelings of love openly. Sometimes you may hide your feelings, while at other times you may exaggerate them to the point that people feel suffocated. This can drive other people away.

To balance the heart chakra, you need to sit with your legs crossed. Touch the tips of your index fingers and thumbs together. Allow your left hand to rest on your knee while holding your right hand in front of the lower part of your breastbone, thumb and index finger together pointing upward. Concentrate on the heart chakra and feel the warmth that spreads from it throughout the body. It shall make you feel cleansed in a while.

The chant for the heart chakra is Yam, pronounced with a rounded sound of, "Yaw-mmm". Although the pronunciation is a bit different, think of when something tastes good or feels good and we tend to say "Yum!" This may bring a smile to your face, which is good because that is what the heart chakra is all about.

The Throat Chakra

Location in the body: just above the top of the breastbone and the base of the throat area.

Color: Blue

Physical associations in the body: thyroid, parathyroid, airways of the throat and upper lungs, the jaw and arms.

Personality aspects: being outspoken, creating true and stable relationships, connection with nature, strength of character through conviction of your words, beliefs and actions; being diplomatic.

Emotional associations: jealousy, regrets and feelings of guilt. Aids you in being compassionate, working with the heart chakra, without feelings of superiority or inferiority to others; not having to compare yourself to others.

Mental associations: health, knowledge and decisiveness. Creativity, especially in professions such as acting, dancing, music, artistry and public speaking. Diplomacy arises out of a healthy throat chakra.

Throat chakra imbalances can cause shy behavior, introversion, confused and inconsistent opinions, self-doubt and several other problems. You can face problems with your creativity and it is possible that you can develop hearing issues. It can also cause you to talk too much or too little. Sometimes, you may say things that make no sense.

Like the sacral chakra, you can bend your knees and sit in the Vajra Asana position to heal this chakra. Hold your hands in front of you at the bottom of the breastbone, palms facing up. Interweave your fingers together on the inside of your hands but leave out the thumbs. Let the tips of your thumbs then touch at the top and extend them, forming a circle between them and your index fingers. Breathe out only through your nostrils. You will feel the vibrations in your skull and this will help to relax you slowly. Envision the throat chakra inside your body as you do this.

The chant for the throat chakra is Ham. This is not pronounced like the meat, it is voiced deeply in the throat with a rounded mouth as, "Haw-mmm".

The Third Eye Chakra

Location in the body: just above the eyes, in between the eyebrows

Color: Indigo

Physical associations in the body: eyes, face, sinuses, nervous system and pituitary gland.

Personality aspects: being very visual, visionary, intuitive for making important decisions in your life. Dissolves conditionings along with bad habits, false ideals, misidentifications and ego, opening us up to a greater awareness.

Nobility and humbleness of the inner spirit, smoothing out the edges of self-expression.

Emotional associations: regulates the ego, helping us to be forgiving and compassionate by letting go of any withheld anger, resentment or hatred against anyone.

Mental associations: being more conscious and aware of your surroundings, of yourself; on a level field, everything in life takes a step up in clarity. Another way to put it is how we become more apt to perceive the subtler context of life in every way. Allows us to explore our inner self, to know what makes us who we are and why we do the things we do. Clears thoughts we've been conditioned into thinking, promoting understanding and allowing you to question things you don't know about or often take for granted.

When the third eye chakra is underactive, it can make a person rely too much on others without forming strong opinions of his or her own. He or she may not be able to make decisions for himself or herself. When overactive, it can tend to make you a daydreamer and an escapist. You may develop cognitive biases and may reject or twist facts to suit your own beliefs. You can even start hallucinating if things get really bad.

To heal this chakra, you have to sit cross-legged and place your hands in front of the lower part of your breast with the palms facing each other but not touching. Start to form this hand gesture with your fingers extended, as it is a bit complicated. Touch the tips of your middle fingers together. Now bend the rest of your fingers inward so that the backs of them are touching from the second knuckle to the tip of the finger. Point your thumbs toward you and touch the top pads of them together. After this, you have to imagine the third eye chakra on your forehead and feel it glowing, as if it is shining light from the spiritual world and connected to the real world. Chant "Om" in a low drone sound, and continue to do this until you feel relaxed and free.

The chant for the third eye chakra is a nice resounding Om, pronounced "Ohh-mmm". As with the other chants, you will want to feel this one right from your diaphragm.

The Crown Chakra

Location in the body: At the top of the head

Color: Violet or white

Physical associations in the body: brain, central nervous system, eyes, pineal gland. Balances all other aspects of your wellbeing from the physical, emotional and mental to the spiritual.

Personality aspects: being conscious and mindful in all areas of life. Integrates all other chakras and melds their qualities into one. Promotes creativity, inspiration and natural attraction.

Emotional associations: inner peace, pure bliss. You feel profound love with no room for prejudice in your heart.

Mental associations: Promotes wisdom; ultimate understanding. Direct connection to the divine. A whole new realm of perception, beyond anything we have ever experienced before with our 5 physical senses. There is an understanding of all humankind as a family; everyone and everything including nature is connected as one living entity, a lot like how the individual cells in your body work together to make a complete, well-functioning person.

Imbalances of the crown chakra can cause people to become rigid and detached from the spiritual world. They find it difficult to be satisfied with anything, and make an issue of the smallest problems. It can make you materialistic, cause headaches, make you indecisive, cause you to overthink, and much more. It can also make you overly spiritual, feeling detached from the real world.

For this chakra, you have to sit with your legs crossed and keep your hands in front of your stomach. Allow your ring fingers to point upward and touch at the top pads. Cross the rest of your fingers as if folding your hands together with the left thumb underneath the right. When you have taken up this position or *mudra*, you have to envision the crown chakra on top of your head and concentrate on it. You can see it as a big lotus flower blooming from your head with it glowing in a vibrant violet light. After this, chant a low drone "Om" sound and let it vibrate throughout your skull. This will make you feel peaceful and will help ease the flow of spiritual energy.

The chant for the crown chakra is Aum and it is pronounced fluidly in three parts, "Ahh-Ohh-mmm"

A great way to practice meditation with the chakras is by visualizing a sort of light passing through your chakras as you meditate. This is the flow of the energy through your subtle system, lighting up your chakras as it goes.

Besides that, you should try to feel grounded and connected to the nature as much as possible. This is because after all, everything is a part of nature. When you feel that you are one with it, your root chakra gets stronger and it is easier for the energy to start flowing through the rest of the body.

Please note that when you are working with the chakras, it is important that you always start with healing the root chakra, since this is your foundational being. Once you feel stable in this area, you can move on to the next one. Each one should be worked subsequently from the next one below it. They should also be worked one at a time, so one per session when you are starting out. By doing this, starting with the root, you are cultivating a strong, powerful foundation for the very basis from which you live and engage in any action.

Sofia Johansson

Chapter 6

7 Day Plan to Combat Fatigue

To effectively combat fatigue, you would have to establish a habit. But we can all agree that drastically changing your lifestyle to combat fatigue can be a challenge. But through this suggested 7-day plan, you can gradually increase your energy levels without making drastic changes to your lifestyle.

Day 1: Take Out Simple Carbs for Breakfast

Many of us are used to eating simple carbs in the morning for breakfast like sugary cereals, caramel lattes, and other fattening baked goodies. The problem with eating such for breakfast is that it gives you an instant boost but also crashes you down quickly. For your first day, take out such food items in your breakfast menu and replace them with complex carbs instead such as whole wheat bread or oatmeal. Both are healthier options that will also help provide you with sustainable energy levels.

Day 2: Eat High-Fiber and High-Protein Snacks

On your second day, add a high-fiber and high-protein snack in your daily menu. Pistachios or dried beans are great to have as snacks. Eat them whenever you feel hungry to keep your body's sugar level regulated and to keep your metabolism running as well.

Day 3: Multivitamins for Energy

Taking in multivitamins in the morning can help supply you with needed energy for the day. Multivitamins contain key nutrients that the body needs to sustain energy and boost the immune system. Make taking multivitamins a habit on this day.

Day 4: Rest

Your goal for day 4 should be that you get at least 8 hours of sleep. Try to manage your time better and make sure that you are in bed on time to have 8 hours of rest. The body takes about 6 to 8 hours to recuperate after a day of activities. This is why if you sleep for less than 6 hours, you feel sluggish and sleepy all day. Your body has not fully recuperated yet and is continuously repairing as you go through your day. Repairing the body takes a lot of energy which is why you feel sleepy and tired. So, make sure to rest for

6-8 hours to make sure that your body has fully recuperated so your energy can be used for accomplishing your work for the day.

Day 5: Hydration

On this day, make sure to count how much water you take. You should have at least 8 glasses of water. Water helps cleanse the body of toxins that can cause fatigue. Moreover, dehydration makes the body malfunction. The cells need water in order for it to function properly. Without water, the cells will not convert and store energy. The result: you feel sluggish, tired, and weak throughout the day. Make sure that you drink enough amounts of water to keep your body functioning properly.

Day 6: 10 Minute Walk

It may seem illogical for some people to keep walking when they already feel tired but physical activity can actually help increase energy levels. On the 6th day, make sure that you do at least 10 minutes of continuous walking as your form of physical activity.

Day 7: Breathing Exercises

On the 7th day, practice some breathing exercises to increase energy levels. This will not only help increase energy levels but also help clear the mind and relieve stress. Try to stay still for at least 10 minutes in one place and clear your mind of everything. Breath deep in and out for 10 minutes and you will feel instantly refreshed and energized after. This is best done early in the morning before you start your day.

This 7-day plan is the start to turning simple activities into a habit so you can feel more energized, happier, and more enthusiastic to face life.

Chapter 7

Eat Your Way to Overcoming Chronic Fatigue

Feeling tired is normal but when it becomes chronic, it can be a sign of more serious illnesses. It has been mentioned in the previous chapter that you have to eat healthy in order to beat fatigue.

Doctors say that there seems to be a lot of people complaining about extreme exhaustion and chronic fatigue, prompting most medical experts to conclude that fatigue is the most common health complaint of people today.

Eat to have energy

In order to restore your energy, you need to eat foods that will boost your energy. Your body needs fuel in order to function well and to ensure your overall well-being.

How you eat

It is also imperative that you eat the right way. What does this mean? If you eat too fast, the stomach does not receive signals from the brain that it is already full. You fail to enjoy your food if you eat too fast. The key is to eat in moderation. Slowly taking meals gives your brain the ability to recognize that you are hungry and that you have already eaten.

It is important to establish eating patterns

Your timing in eating your meals is just as important as what you put in your mouth. You will feel sluggish every time after a full meal, especially when you ate more than you usually do. The body will need to exert more effort to digest the big meal, and this will require the use of energy. To avoid this, it is recommended that you eat smaller meal portions throughout the day. Eating six small meals a day is recommended.

No to processed food

While a huge hamburger and a side of fries can boost your energy, they are too oily. They may satisfy your hunger but not for long and soon you'll be craving for more. Processed foods, liked packaged foods, canned goods, and processed meats with high sodium contents are full of chemicals that your body does not need. Excess sodium in your body can actually slow you down.

Add more fresh fruits and vegetables

You stand to get more nutrients from fresh foods and they are easier to digest. The brighter and more colorful the fruits and vegetables, the healthier they are. Raspberries, blueberries, and tomatoes are perfect. Carrots, broccoli, spinach, and oranges will also boost your energy.

Stay away from caffeine

Drinking coffee may perk you up a little, especially during the first few sips, but doctors say that this sudden perk doesn't last long. After an energy rush, you will also crash quite suddenly. Avoid drinking coffee to stabilize your energy.

Avoid energy drinks

Energy drinks are quite popular these days. Like sodas, these energy drinks might be able to give you an adrenaline rush but not for long. Besides, these drinks are sugary so it is not recommended that you consume these in large numbers. You do not get any nutritional benefits from these beverages.

Add more lean proteins to your diet

Avoid red meat because it contains more fat that takes too long to digest. Choose lean meat instead as your protein source. When you eat chicken, it is important that you do take out the skin before cooking. Eat fish like salmon because of its high omega-3 fatty acid content. A hardboiled egg is a good source of protein, too.

Foods rich in iron

Iron is not just for anemia. Low levels of iron in the body cause the red blood cells to find other sources of oxygen. Low iron content results in poor energy, too.

Choose whole grains and starches

Refined sugars and carbohydrates do not have nutritional benefits. You have to admit it, though: you consume more of these than the healthier alternatives. Whole grains and complex carbohydrates can help boost energy. As mentioned earlier, sugar should be avoided. Whole grain cereals are also perfect.

Stay away from the "whites"

White bread, white potatoes, white pasta, and white rice have high glycemic index. These foods trigger the development of hypoglycemia or decreased blood sugar levels. Hypoglycemia has fatigue as one of its symptoms. Whole grains are recommended.

White potatoes may be substituted by sweet potatoes while white rice can be replaced with brown rice. These are healthier as they contain more vitamins and minerals.

Eat nuts

If you want snacks or something to munch on, choose nuts. They can boost your energy. The best sources of nutrients are Brazil nuts, cashew nuts, walnuts, hazelnuts, and pecan. Eating them raw is recommended.

Drink lots of water

Do away with sodas and coffee, drink water instead.

It helps to add food supplements

Taking food supplements in addition to eating the right kinds of foods ensures that you are getting the appropriate vitamins and minerals your body needs. Ask your doctors what is best for you consume before purchasing these.

The following nutrients might be beneficial:

Vitamin C

Vitamin D

Folic acid

L-carnithine

Zinc

Essential fatty acids

Milk

Alkalize your body

One of the general disorders that fatigue is often an indicator for is a weak immune system. Patients show high levels of white blood cells that react by causing inflammation, along with unusually low levels of the killer T cells that fight off infection and pathogens.

Inflammation, the prominence of bad bacteria in the body, Candida, viruses, cancer and pathogens all have one thing in common involving the body: their ability to survive in an alkaline environment goes to zero. You have probably heard about the body's pH levels before and how they should be just above the neutral pH of water at 7 (the body is primarily made up of water, making dehydration a serious issue). On either side of the neutral 7 pH, 1-6 being acidic and 8-14 being alkaline. Every living and non-living thing has a pH, so what we put in our bodies affects our own pH levels.

Studies have shown that bacteria and cancer cannot survive in alkaline environments. Thus, with an alkaline diet you will already be healing and preventing your body from taking on further illness. Pathogens and the like thrive however in acidic environments. The standard and unsubstantial diet of fast and junk foods, which is nearly everything that isn't found at a restaurant that values the quality of its food or food markets that are health conscious, all contributes to a sloth-induced state of functioning that catches up to you over time, from the physical to the mental to the emotional.

Here is a general list of what turns our body into an acidic environment:

Spicy foods

Fatty foods

Dairy

Sugar

Simple carbs, which turn into sugar when digested

Acidic foods like orange juice and coffee

Tobacco products

Here is a general list of what turns our body into an alkaline environment:

Lots of filtered or alkaline water

Root vegetables: turnip, carrot, parsnip, sweet potatoes, beet, radish, onion

Dark, green, leafy vegetables: romaine lettuce, spinach, kale, collard greens, broccoli

Baking soda: find a baking soda that states it contains no aluminum on the packaging, as aluminum is a heavy metal that can be harmful to the body. Start with a teaspoon and stir into a tall glass of water. Sip, do not gulp. Drink one of these daily to a couple times per week. Make sure you do so on an *empty stomach*, either in the morning before you have eaten anything or at least four hours since your last meal. Otherwise, you will feel bloated and the effect will not be as potent.

Vinegars: it's true that vinegars are acidic, however they are effective in raising the body's alkalinity levels because they are less acidic than your stomach juices.

o   Apple cider vinegar: make sure that it says "with the MOTHER" on the label. This is a kind of yeast that is very good for the entire digestive system of the body. Drink one ounce of apple cider vinegar daily or a couple times per week (with a chaser, if you prefer).

o   Balsamic vinegar: Great to put on your salads, there are several delicious vinaigrette recipes that use balsamic vinegar as a base. Combine with a dark leafy green salad and you've just given yourself a power boost.

Turmeric: you can consider this to be a gem spice. There have been books written on turmeric and its beneficial effects for the body. It is not so much an alkalizer for the body as it is an anti-inflammatory. Turmeric will free your stomach and lower intestines from any heavy or undigested food particles. It has also been noted that when combined with what must be *coarse ground* black pepper, turmeric's properties are absorbed by the body by 400 times more. Listed below are some of its conventional uses.

Sprinkle on baked, pan-fried, roasted or grilled meats

Eggs w/ black pepper & chives

Stir-fry dishes

Steamed vegetables

Golden milk: it's a strange name, but your taste buds will be easily swayed. Consider it to be a milky version of a potent tea. You can easily find a recipe by searching for the name online. You can also read more about the powerful effects of turmeric there.

8 Foods That Could Help You Gain More Energy

Food also plays an essential role in combating fatigue. Food is actually where we get our energy from. The calories contained in food are converted into energy so we can perform our daily tasks.

Here are some foods you need to eat more of so that you can have more energy every day.

Eggs – the yolks in the egg contain high amounts of B vitamins that help boost the energy production of the body. Vitamin B is also responsible in converting the food we eat into energy. Eggs are also rich in D vitamin that helps maintain strong bones. Furthermore, eggs are probably the best sources of protein that is essential to help the body recuperate after doing strenuous activities so you maintain energy levels. Expert Tip: stick to one whole egg plus 2-3 egg whites for a satisfying breakfast minus too much cholesterol and fat.

Edamame – edamame or soybeans are rich in nutrients that boost energy levels such as B vitamins, copper, and phosphorous. B vitamins as discussed above help breakdown the carbohydrates in the body to be converted into energy. Copper and phosphorous on the other hand are both responsible for converting food into energy and storing it in the cells so energy is readily available when needed. Just one cup serving of this a day is already enough as it is already packed with 8g of fiber and 17g or protein.

Whole Grain Oats – whole grain oats and cereals helps slow down the release of glucose into the bloodstream so energy levels are sustained throughout the day. Glucose is the sugar found in the blood that is converted into energy. If the process of releasing glucose into the bloodstream is slowed down, your body won't experience an initial high and then suddenly crash down later because there is no more glucose to be converted into energy. Eat whole grain oats and cereals instead for breakfast so energy levels are sustained until your next meal.

Trail Mix for Snacks – nuts mixed with dried fruits make for a great snack as it contains the ideal mixture of healthy fats, protein and fiber. Just like whole grains, nuts and dried fruits also slow down the release of glucose into the bloodstream to be converted into energy so there is constant and steady supply of energy. Protein also helps slow down the metabolism of carbohydrates and helps repair muscles that are damaged after performing strenuous activities. Fats in nuts are also known to help provide a long term supply of energy that can last for hours. Because carbohydrates are the first that the body converts into energy, it is easily depleted. Once carbohydrates supply is fully consumed, the body relies on fats for energy.

Drink lots of water – dehydration is one of the early signs of lack of energy. Dehydration actually happens much sooner than starvation which is why you need to drink more water. Water helps cleanse the body of toxins that can cause fatigue. Without enough water in the body, the cells will not function properly in converting food into energy. The result: fatigue and lethargy. This is why drinking lots of water every day is important in sustaining energy levels. If you workout, drink water before heading out for your activity.

Quinoa – quinoa is probably one of the healthiest grains you can ever find out there. Aside from containing lots of protein, it is also gluten-free. Quinoa is also known to contain high amounts of essential amino acids, lysine, methionine, and cysteine that are all ideal nutrients for a post-workout meal to help the muscles recuperate and sustain energy levels. Other nutrients found in quinoa include folate, magnesium, phosphorous and manganese that are all responsible for providing and sustaining energy levels.

Pumpkin Seeds – a handful of roasted pumpkin seeds or raw seeds can give you that jolt of power and strength needed in a workout. It is a great source of fiber, protein, and various healthy fats to help you feel full and energized as you workout. It is also a good source of magnesium, manganese, zinc, and phosphorus that provide added energy.

Goji Berries – this has long been used in Chinese medicine to help boost energy levels and normalize the release of hormones. Goji berries are also known to help enhance the overall mood of a person, enable you to handle stress better, and boost the mind and memory retention. It is also known to help promote better blood circulation so nutrients are equally distributed throughout the body providing you with more energy.

Eating the right foods can certainly help increase energy levels and fight fatigue.

Sofia Johansson

Conclusion

Thank you again for downloading this book!

Fatigue may seem like a phantom vampire, unseen and ever-present, draining you of the energy from doing all the things that you need to do and love to do in your life. It doesn't have to be that way. Although there are so many people out there who are experiencing similar problems such as yourself and there are many reasons for it, the most commonly occurring reasons for excessive fatigue stem from lifestyle choices. Now you have a better understanding as to which kinds of lifestyle choices contribute to fatigue symptoms and which help to relieve you from fatigue.

Sometimes all a lifestyle change requires is a little knowledge and nudge in the right direction to apply it. Ultimately though, it will always be up to ourselves to make those better decisions because no one else is going to force us or do it for us. Only when we have absolutely had enough as we will allow ourselves to have in leading a compromising lifestyle do we find the courage and motivation to do something about it. Many times that built-up drive and passion breaks through the heavy blanket of lethargy in a short burst that will bring us out to the gym for the first couple weeks of the new year or eating healthily for a month or two until we go back to our old routine. By then, the passion wears out because we have only been driven by our external circumstances and the push to move forward has lessened once we answer it.

To establish an enduring state of living that feeds back into your efforts and amplifies them, assuring that your energy wheels keep turning, the focus should be not only on exerting this drive and passion sitting within you, coming from whatever reason. It should question, "How do I keep the passion going? How can I call upon it whenever I need it and carry myself steadily and confidently in times that I don't?" It becomes a matter of cultivating your own internal energy system and training it to work for you on a regular basis at a slow and steady pace – your pace.

Start with small steps, make consistency a cornerstone of your process, and focus on integrating your life with practices that give you back energy. Any and all of the practices that have been provided for you in this book alone can be practiced from 5 minutes in the day to 10, 30, or an hour. It should be no problem to find pockets of time such as these throughout your day to engage in energy-replenishing activities, no matter how busy you are. If you are not able to fit an hour of time into your day to give back to yourself, then you may wish to seriously question your lifestyle and what it *is* doing for you. This is *your* life. You get to choose how you live it. Just remember that life is never a matter about *finding* time to do things. You must *make* time for it. If it is truly important to you, you will.

I hope this is the start of a new life for you — a life that is free from stress and exhaustion. You will begin to enjoy life as soon as you practice the things you have learned from this book. Also, don't forget to share with your friends and loved ones what you have learned so that they do not let fatigue ruin their otherwise happy and healthy lives.

Check Out My Other Books

Below you'll find some of my other popular books that are popular on Amazon and Kindle as well. I have added some other books from fellow authors in order to support their job too.

Simply search them on Amazon Kindle by the Title below to check them out. Alternatively, you can visit my author page on Amazon to see other work done by me.

- **Time Management Made Easy!**

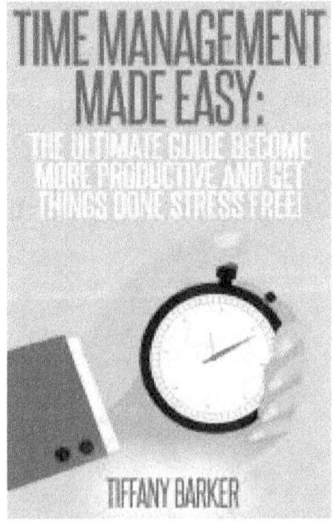

Master the clock with this guide, Tiffany has put on this title her best techniques to become more productive and getting things done stress free!

- **Influence and Charisma: Build Rapport, Develop Your Interpersonal Skills and Learn The Secrets of Power Negotiating**

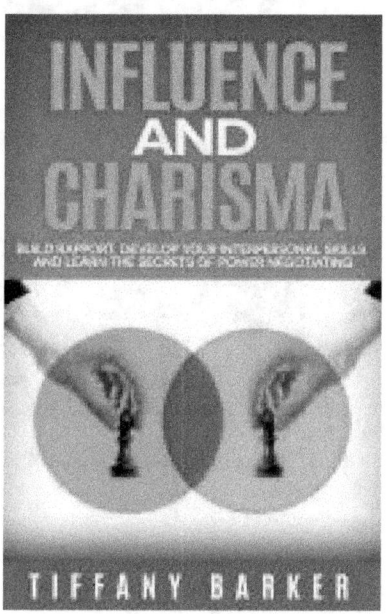

Tiffany won't teach you how to manipulate nor abuse to other people but how to be a positive influence with a high sense of ethic.

- **Leadership Game Plan**

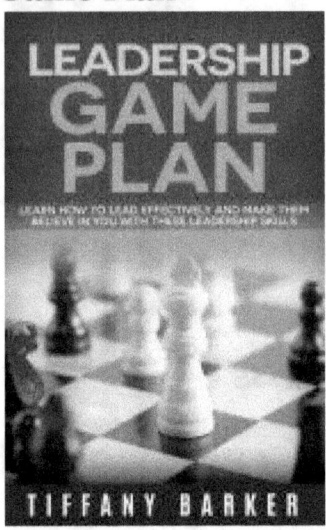

Make them believe in you with the leadership skills that Tiffany is going to teach you in this title!

www.ingramcontent.com/pod-product-compliance
Lightning Source LLC
Chambersburg PA
CBHW071214280526
45787CB00002B/681